Walking Through Fog
A Christian Perspective on Fibromyalgia

kate gibson

Copyright © 2016 kate gibson

All rights reserved.

ISBN: 1517184541
ISBN-13: 978-1517184544

DEDICATION

To my very own
Red Panda—Jon Gibson

CONTENTS

	Introduction	i
1	Recovering Identity	1
2	Embracing Vulnerability	4
3	Facing the Darkness	7
4	Choosing Treatments	12
5	Fighting the Pain	17
6	Celebrating the Victories	20
7	Inevitable Relapse	23
8	Living Today	26
9	Shifting Relationships	29
10	Moving Forward	32

INTRODUCTION

"We heard you were feeling sick today. Hope you get well soon!" I can't tell you how disheartening these words have been to me over the past few years since diagnosis. I know they are said in full sincerity, but somehow that doesn't make it any easier hearing it the tenth time and knowing that it means one more person doesn't understand the word "chronic" in your chronic disease. They don't seem to understand the constant struggle to be presentable or go to the store. They seem to take for granted that you will function normally.

If you're picking up this book because you know someone with a chronic condition, and you're starting to feel guilty for telling them to "get well soon," please don't. Without friends like you in our lives, we would be missing a lot. Here's a suggestion. Maybe the next time you feel at a loss for what to say but want to be supportive, you could try something like, "I'm sorry you feel so horrible. I'm happy to hang out with you, whether we go out or just sit on the couch." Or perhaps a simple "I'm sorry you are in pain. I don't really know what to say or how to help, but I'm here, and I care."

Believe it or not, sometimes we don't want to be told to look on the bright side or that "things aren't so bad" or to "think of someone who has it worse." Sometimes we just need someone to empathize with us, even when they can't make it better. Letting us be honest with where we're at does make it a little better. Whatever your reason for picking up this book (whether patient or caregiver), I hope you find it encouraging and helpful. So without further introduction, let's get to it. Enjoy!

1 RECOVERING IDENTITY

People find their identities in a variety of places. Some pour themselves into their work, becoming the best in their field. Others invest in family putting everything they have into their closest relationships to be the best Mom, Dad, Nana, or Papa. No matter what area of life it is, people have a tendency to find their identity in something they do—whether it is how well they work, how faithfully they serve others, or how deeply they love.

Church is no exception to this rule. People are constantly referred to by the role they play in the church or greater Christian community. Pastors, missionaries, teachers, evangelists, organists, and even nursery workers can be defined by the role they fulfill at church.

When you live in a culture that thinks this way, it can be easy to start seeing your life in these terms. What I do equals who I am, which equals what I'm worth. This might tentatively work with someone in the position of Senior Pastor of a large church. But what happens when you apply this same philosophy to someone in chronic pain who struggles to leave the house once a week to even attend Sunday morning's service?

It soon becomes a big problem when you have a chronic illness. It doesn't matter how much you want to, you just cannot fill the roles in your community that you once did. You can't teach that class of junior high girls or lead that women's Bible study. You can barely get food together for your family much less bring covered dishes to church. They can forget asking you to chase around the children in the nursery three times a month, because you're struggling to get around your own house.

In a work setting, it's easy to feel your identity slowly being ripped from you as you just can't work up the energy to work late anymore. Those large stacks of files that you used to be able to catch up on for everyone else just get away from you now. You're supposed to be the one reliable worker that your boss can count on when everyone else bails on them. Now you are so tired and in pain you sit at your desk and want to cry.

This leads to additional performance reviews as your memory starts to fail in the fast-paced work environment you used to thrive in. The coworkers who used to depend on you to cover for them are now annoyed that the work they dumped on your desk is still sitting there untouched, burying the work you were supposed to get done beforehand.

At home you feel like a failure with your spouse or your children. Just leaving home to get to work in the morning takes all the energy you have. By the time you get home at night, you can barely move enough to get to the couch and crash.

You used to be the friend that always had time to listen when someone in your group had a problem. You could give them the warmest hugs with the best advice, but now you're too busy and too sick to even respond to their messages. You're afraid to make plans with anyone, because what if you get too sick and have to cancel on them last minute?

Gradually you feel your life closing in on you as the stress builds and builds. The walls feel as if they are growing closer, and just seeing certain people's faces on your Caller ID gives you a tight feeling in your chest from the stress of having to talk with them.

You feel trapped, and you wonder what happened to the identity you worked so hard to build up that made everyone around you like you? Where is the person your husband fell in love with? Where is the employee your boss was clamoring to promote? Where is the church member your pastor was praising for faithfulness? Where is the friend who never let the others down?

You are just not that person anymore. Your new identity: Sick. Inconvenient. Helpless. Useless. Burden on Society. Unreliable. You have become the person you can't stand. The person that other people make allowances for, but talk about behind their back. The person who can't help because they're "less than."

It is a crushing blow to feel your identity being torn from your very soul and replaced with a crinkled shell of who you used to be. It brings grief and mourning, and some people never make it past that. I have been there. I have gazed at the life I thought I would have, and the life I now know will never come, and yes, I have grieved for it. But that is not the end, because I know something about identity I haven't shared yet. It's something I have to remind myself of every time I start to grieve again over the future that will never be.

Our identity is not tied to what we do, and it never was. Nobody can define us based on an illness or a hobby or even our relationships, because there is one thing that defines my identity—Jesus Christ. Because of the value that Jesus created in me as a human being and saw again on the cross as worth repurchasing at great cost, I have value. I have value whether I am in Haiti feeding starving orphans or sitting on the couch in our apartment under a blanket writhing in pain. God does not define me by the list of activities I'm involved in at church, the number of well-paying jobs I've held, or even the picture perfect family I raise. He defines me by the inherent value He created in humanity. He views me through the completion He brought to me by taking my sin and offering me a loving relationship with Him.

I may feel as though I have lost my identity, but the truth is—this is step one in finding it. I may feel as though I am only a weaker shell of myself, but the truth is—that facing reality without hiding has made me stronger than ever. I may think my life is over, but the truth is—it has just begun.

2 EMBRACING VULNERABILITY

Nobody likes feeling vulnerable. We are taught from a young age to keep that "stiff upper lip." For some reason it's frowned upon to have weakness and even more so to show it in public. It could be from a number of factors. We could blame it on competitive workplaces, gossiping churches, movies, and TV shows that show us how to bottle our feelings and forget about them. However, it doesn't really matter where the message originated from, because it's just not a workable solution for someone with chronic disease plaguing them on a daily basis.

You may be able to hide the fact that you feel like a prisoner in your own body from yourself and those around you for a while, but it will only be a matter of time before you can't hide your physical weaknesses anymore. You may start slowing down or your memory might fail you at the wrong moment. Whatever your specific vulnerability is; rest assured, it's coming if it hasn't already. The question is not how do we avoid it; the question becomes how do we deal with it?

For those of us with chronic conditions, vulnerability is a way of life, often both physically and emotionally. Pain takes a toll on our emotions and leaves us weary before we've even gotten out of bed in the morning. We already live with our vulnerability tied around our neck like a noose, so what are we going to do with it?

We could try to follow the lead from the rest of healthy society that just buries it as deep as it can and then runs from the hole until it shoots back to the surface. We could go into denial until everyone around us is confronting us about it. Or, we could just embrace it. Yes, I said we should embrace our vulnerability. How does this work? Glad you asked.

If we acknowledge to ourselves that we have deep vulnerability that we can't get rid of, what are we really giving up? Our pride? Our sense of security? Make that *false* security. The truth is, everyone is vulnerable in some way, even healthy people. What's incredibly sad is that even within the church (which should be the safest place on earth to admit vulnerability) people are afraid to admit they are weak and broken and hurting. Instead of coming to church to honestly share our sorrows and pain with each other, we pull ourselves together to present a front so the church people will think we're spiritual. We can't possibly have them pity us if they realize we are a mess, or worse—judge us for it.

Before my fibromyalgia got worse, I used to view friendship as something I entered from a position of strength. I looked around at my peers and tried to find people I felt I could get along with and appear strong in front of. I wanted people with whom I shared areas of strength. I was drawn into friendships with people who could appreciate, or at the very least endure, my sense of humor, musical abilities, and eccentric academic pursuits. We might be "friends," but likely we only discussed topics that made us both feel comfortable.

The problem came once my condition grew increasingly worse. I found that I no longer could approach friendship from a position of strength. I could no longer look for people who shared my areas of talent, skill, and dedication. Even some friends I'd known for years fell away gradually. I found that I now came to the table with no positions of strength left, only vulnerability.

But a beautiful thing happened. In losing my ability to keep up with people who shared my strengths, I gained a deep appreciation for the ones who were willing to share in my vulnerability. I gained time to sit and listen to the vulnerability of others, and suddenly friendship was not so much about finding people on equal footing with me, as it was about finding people who would share my weakness and would let me share in theirs. We could encourage each other, because we knew the struggles we were facing, and we didn't have to pretend we were both ok.

It's easy as Christians to look for friends who share our skills and interests and only talk about things that make us look strong and confident. But it's just possible that sometimes we need to embrace the vulnerabilities that God has given us so that we can share those with others and find a deeper connection than something we're both good at. Some of the best conversations I have been able to have in the past few years have involved shared deeply painful and personal details of my struggle with someone else and letting them know that they are not alone in their fight. They are not alone in their pain.

If the only thing I have in common with my friends and family is what I am good at, then when I struggle and I hurt (and you know you will) I will struggle and hurt alone. No one has been allowed to share in my vulnerability. We must stop being afraid of our weakness and begin embracing the human frailty that God has given to us. Either way, we're going to have it. We might as well use it the way He wants us to.

3 FACING THE DARKNESS

Before you enter this chapter, I should warn you about something. **This chapter will be primarily discussing both chronic anxiety and clinical depression.** These are not topics that I take lightly, and hopefully that will be clear in the paragraphs to follow. The reason I am telling you this in advance is to prepare you for what you're about to read.

Anxiety and depression are not easy topics to wade though. For this reason, I think it is important for you to be willing to mentally engage with what I have to share before proceeding any further. If you need to read the rest of this book and come back at the end, go ahead. Just be sure that when you enter this chapter, you are in a frame of mind to engage with some heavier thoughts. With that disclaimer stated, let's dive into this.

With topics such as these, it can be difficult to know where to begin. There are so many possible angles to approach it from. Because I am coming from experience and not in the role of a detached expert, I will approach it the way I know best—the way we become acquainted with it in real life—through experiencing it.

I have experienced some level of anxiety my entire life. Even as a child I was prone to unhelpful cycles of obsessive thinking. I was not the kid who could be distracted from her fears by something shiny or a piece of candy. Though I didn't realize it at the time, I was developing thought patterns as a young child that would later result in destructive thinking as a young adult. Whether it was severe social anxiety, nonstop worrying about hypothetical burglars breaking into our house and shooting everyone, or something else equally paralyzing, I tried to hold it in my head and act like nothing was bothering me.

I was able to cope pretty well for a while. It wasn't until I reached high school that I began to feel hopeless and frustrated. I began feeling a building pressure in my mind. On occasion the mental and emotional struggle going on in my head would lead me to act out self-destructively. I didn't really understand why, but I found some amount of relief from punching walls until my knuckles felt raw or hitting my head against hard surfaces. It was all just to stop the internal chaos. I should note at this point that this was not a healthy coping mechanism. I am simply describing what I was doing, not condoning that behavior.

The head banging and self-harm of punching walls, doors, or even trees continued into my college days. As stress built up in my mind, I still found no strength to fight back, and I was afraid to ask for help. Good Christians didn't hurt themselves. Reasonable people didn't hurt themselves. At the time I didn't realize I was engaging in self-harm behavior. I just knew I needed some relief from the mental anguish. I decided not to think about why I was doing it, and I made sure to hide it as well as I could at my Christian college.

I should probably explain at this point that when I say anxiety, I don't mean the type of fear that you can simply decide to disregard. I am talking about mental bombardment that seemingly comes from nowhere and makes it difficult to breathe. This anxiety produces an elevated heart rate, circular frantic thinking, and physical exhaustion. It feels like quicksand. The harder you fight to get out, the deeper it pulls you down. Eventually you are just trying to physically hold onto something to get yourself through the roughest nights.

As a Christian I believe there has been some aspect of spiritual warfare involved in my anxiety, though I would not go so far as to say it's always involved. Sometimes, my brain just gets stuck on a cycle. It's like a record getting caught in a groove and repeating the same thing until you can't take it anymore. In my brain it seemed as if there were no option of taking the needle off that groove. It was doomed to repeat until it eventually damaged the record or ran out of power.

This cycle, if left unchecked for an extended period of time, can easily lead to depression. Your mind and body can only handle living in "fight or flight" mode for so long without becoming worn out. After your limit is reached and exceeded, the next stage is often giving up hope that things will ever change or be controlled.

Once you have felt the anxiety of your body falling apart beyond control without explanation, it is not difficult to imagine that hope will become impossible to hold onto. It's all too easy to slip into believing that life will always be as hard as it is now or that things will just get worse. It's a dangerous direction to move in, though, because hope and normalcy often become elusive once you've stopped fighting for them.

I have struggled with this deadly combination of anxiety and bouts of depression off and on for years. I thought I could just believe more, try harder, and decide more passionately to fight it, but I failed every time. I kept coming to a point where erratic thoughts and scary ideas started bombarding my mind.

I started getting counseling from a trusted advisor through my church, and I thought this would be enough to get me back on track where everyone else in my life seemed to be—mentally stable at the very least. I expected to be told that I was in some sin that was causing the mental and spiritual turmoil. I wasn't prepared to delve deeply into exactly what I was experiencing. It would be an understatement to say that I was thoroughly shocked at the eventual suggestion and requirement that I consult my doctor about medication options.

I wrestled with this extensively. I did not want to be one of "those people" who needed meds to deal with life. I didn't want to admit it was a big deal or that I had let it go so far. But having asked God to fix it any other way and after consulting with my husband and counselor, as well as a few close friends who knew my struggle—I finally relented and sought help from my doctor.

Once I explained what was going on in my brain—the thoughts that were assaulting my mind, the uncontrollable cycles of frantic thinking, the blindsiding panic attacks, and the inevitable depression at the end of each cycle—my doctor listened empathetically and agreed that medication was necessary. We agreed on a small dose of *Cymbalta*, which would help with the chronic pain and the cyclical thinking, and a small dose of *Buspar*, which would help prevent the panic attacks.

I was still skeptical, but by this point I was so desperate for something to help that I followed the regimen to the letter. Then I waited to see what would happen. I expected bizarre side effects—feeling numb like a zombie, having even crazier thoughts than before, or hallucinations. Instead, what happened surprised me yet again.

I began to feel control over what I thought about. If frantic thoughts came into my mind unheeded, instead of feeling helpless to cut it off, I finally had the choice to stop. It felt like a miracle. The thoughts might still come, but now I had the power to choose to trust God would work things out. I could decide to stop replaying decisions or fears endlessly in my mind. I also found that knowing I could stop the cyclical thinking made me better able to endure the pain and feel less tense.

I don't mean to imply that the medicine numbed my emotions. On the contrary, I still felt the normal emotions of fear, pain, sadness, joy, happiness, etc. But for the first time in my life I could get sad about events in my life without being afraid of the thoughts that would follow. It was a fantastic feeling.

It has been over a year since I first started taking *Cymbalta*. I am so grateful that my counselor insisted I consult my doctor. It has made a huge difference in my ability to function on a daily basis. While it hasn't completely eliminated problems with my thinking, it has given me a choice to make healthy decisions and choose to think in healthy ways. That is a huge change that you almost have to experience to truly appreciate.

I liken it to adding a STOP/EJECT button to the VCR of my mind. Before there was no button for it; when I reached the end, the tape would automatically rewind itself and start playing again. The only way to find relief was to push PAUSE for short moments or run out of power. Pushing stop and changing tapes is a huge thing.

What I have shared in this chapter is my own experience. I don't have all the answers, and I'm no expert on these topics. This is a process, and I am still fighting most days to make good choices and keep my perspective intact. The only thing I have to offer is empathetic advice.

If any of my words seem familiar to you—if you have ever sat and considered doing something drastic to make the pressure go away, you're not alone in this fight. There are so many people on this journey with you. You may not know them personally, but I am here to tell you that you do not need to face this darkness by yourself.

If you have ever been afraid of the frantic thoughts that bombard your mind and kept silent because you felt you were going crazy—you're not the only person who has experienced it, and it does not make you crazy. It doesn't make you one of "those people." It means that it's time to admit there's a serious problem, and you need help to figure it out.

I know how hard it can be to take this step, because I have done it. I never imagined that I would need this type of help, and I thought it was a "great idea" for "someone else." It's a whole new thought when it becomes you. Take the step if you need it. It will be difficult. You will probably be misunderstood and possibly deeply hurt by people in your life who disapprove, but this is the type of help you can't afford to skip because others won't understand or agree.

Get the help you need, and don't be afraid to make other people uncomfortable with the choices that you make to pursue healthy mental stability. Doctors and medicines that work on the brain are not the enemy. Medications like *Cymbalta* can be just one more weapon in a fight against the real enemy. It may be a rough road, but it's one worth following. The difference is worth the trial and error.

4 CHOOSING TREATMENTS

If you've had fibro for any amount of time, you are no doubt aware of the myriad of treatment options offered both on and off the internet. It seems that anybody with $12 and a label-maker can buy their own website domain name and start bottling their own "miracle fibromyalgia cure" to save the world. In fact, I would be willing to bet if you googled the term "miracle fibromyalgia cure" online, you would find no shortage of results. This is the case with many conditions, but sadly, fibromyalgia tends to attract more than its fair share of "miracle cures." Why is that? Why are patients with fibromyalgia more of a target than some other conditions? I have a few possible answers to that.

I believe some of the size disparity comes from traditional medicine not being able to solidify one particular cause. As long as doctors are unsure of the exact cause of fibromyalgia, the online "experts" are free to give their opinions, and who can prove them wrong? Another, perhaps more disheartening, cause for this free-for-all flows from the fact that since there is no one specifically known cause, there is also no known cure. The symptoms vary from patient to patient, and treatment includes finding ways to ease symptoms for the individual patient.

Because of this admitted lack of objective answers from the authoritative medical community, the online marketplace is free to sell their wares to exhausted, sick patients desperate for some relief that will be permanent. This leads to alternative/natural remedies springing up all across the world claiming to have the definitive cure for fibromyalgia.

For my part, I find this highly unlikely, since the number of people suffering from fibromyalgia worldwide is so high that if anyone had truly discovered a legitimate cure, it would be on international news for weeks on end. Millions of people around the world would be celebrating, and it wouldn't just work for a couple hundred people who found a website and paid their $19.99 plus shipping and handling.

For that reason, I am skeptical about anyone who claims they have found the "cure for fibro" or even the "definitive test" to diagnose it. Either of these discoveries would be so huge, we would be hearing about it on mainstream news for weeks, if not months.

Having made that statement, I do not discount the benefits of trying alternative treatments. It is true that in some cases traditional medicine does not have an answer yet. Fibromyalgia is one of those grey areas that stands on the line between the two fields. Depending on your doctor, you may be able to get all of your symptoms under control and go back to living a relatively normal life. On the other hand, you may have a very difficult time finding a doctor who even acknowledges that fibromyalgia is a big deal. I can see value in pursuing either route or a combination of both.

Personally, I have chosen to follow a more traditional medical journey. I see my regular doctor every few months, and she checks up on how my medications are helping. She also helps advise me on any concerns I have, and we work together to come up with a plan that I am comfortable with. She does not try to force drugs on me for a commission, and she does not try to convince me to follow treatment plans I feel hesitant about. She is one of several advisors I listen to when constructing my own personal healthcare regimen.

In the course of treating my whole array of symptoms, my doctor and I have tried several different types of medications to see what is most effective for me. Among those are drugs in the anti-seizure class (*Gabapentin*, *Tomamax*, etc.), more traditional antidepressants (such as *Amitriptyline*), and medicines that treat a variety of conditions but have proven useful to fight my fibro (Duloxetine, Buspirone, and *Fioricet*).

Gabapentin proved to be a mainstay for nearly a year, but these days I am finding Duloxetine (*Cymbalta*) and Butalbital/Acetaminophen/Caffeine (*Fioricet* or *Esgic*) to be a great team in fighting my pain, specifically headaches. Buspirone (*Buspar*) is an anti-anxiety medication that I have periodically found effective as well.

I also purchased a wearable TENS unit on the internet that I have found extremely helpful for muscle and joint pain as well as helping me sleep more productively at night. My doctor was supportive of that decision, and we incorporated that into my pain management plan.

My point is that I realize there are reasonable arguments for and against traditional medicine, and I personally have tried both traditional and alternative options. I currently take what I find helpful from each side and leave the rest. I don't take medication just to take medication, but if it is truly helpful and not just masking symptoms that need to be noticed, I am not opposed to taking drugs to make life more manageable.

Treatment choices are not easy for anyone, and they get exponentially more difficult when other people disregard your choices and assert their own opinions instead. It can be difficult to admit to your family that your condition necessitates a steady dosage of anti-depressants or a temporary use of anti-anxiety medications. That shouldn't stop you from using them if that is what you and your doctor decide to use.

It is up to you to take responsibility for your treatment plan and own it. Make a decision by discussing it with your doctor, your spouse, your counselor, your best friends, or whomever you trust with that type of situation. Just make sure to gather advice and make a decision you are comfortable with moving forward. It is not your family's decision, and it is not your church's decision. It's not even your friends' decision. It is a decision that you have to make; although if you are married, your spouse should definitely get input on it as well.

Once you have made the best possible decision for your particular situation, you should stand by it. Other people may not understand, or they may make you feel uncomfortable simply by just making jokes or saying insensitive things about it. You need to stand by your choices. You are not responsible to change their mind, and you are not responsible to make sure your choices in healthcare make them feel better. Be the adult and own your decision. Sometimes that means choosing not to discuss your choice with family members you know will disapprove or friends you know will not understand from previous generic conversations. That's ok. You're not required to disclose your personal medical choices with everyone you know. It is up to you whether you want to tell other people about it or not.

One thing I've noticed in regard to the chronically ill community (primarily online since most of us can't leave our houses to meet in person) is that when you discuss symptoms, we can all agree they are not fun. However, when you start discussing treatment options, sometimes things get a bit controversial, for lack of a better word.

In some forums, it's completely acceptable to discuss differing opinions on what works best for certain symptoms. However, there are some groups where emotions run high and tension grows thick if you start to argue for your chiropractor over someone else's homeopathic expert. They might even get upset, because someone else is simultaneously promoting a miracle cream they purchase from Dr. So-and-so's online clinic based out of Oklahoma. Everyone on that particular forum, however, can band together to cast out the healthcare snob who dared to enter their forum and talk about how happy they are with their traditional doctor and the prescription medications they've been taking. How offensive can you get?

Obviously I'm being a bit facetious here, but the point still stands. While we can all agree that our treatment options are personal, agonizing decisions over which our families have no control, sometimes we lose our reasoning abilities in online conversations regarding the same ideals and principles. Simply put, I think whatever treatment or remedies you find helpful in your struggle with this awful condition are all right with me. I may not agree with the route you choose to take in getting functional (note I did not say "getting well"), but I will support your right to choose that for yourself.

I think we would be better off as a chronically ill community if we stood together under the unified idea that the body and mind are still a mystery to us, and we can't fully explain why we are the way we are. We can agree to disagree on practical methods, while still embracing our community of suffering. We can unite in the name of encouraging each other to keep pursuing wellness in mind and body. That is a cause we can all agree on.

So, while there will be options that work for others but don't do anything for you, it would go a long way to civilize the conversation if we stopped accusing each other's caregivers of conspiracies. No, not all doctors are insensitive pill-pushers who disregard patients in pain for the money from pharmaceutical companies. And no, not everyone offering alternative treatments is a scam artist trying to make easy money off of hurting, desperate people looking for answers. Is it not possible that the truth is somewhere in the middle? There are good people working on both sides of this issue, and there are scams and evil people working on both sides as well. The goal is not to point fingers at the "other side" but to continue looking for something helpful and hopefully find a community of friends along the way. We may find that one side supplies everything we need, or we may find we need a combination.

Either way, the answer is not found in mudslinging or in proclaiming ourselves the expert on our condition. We are merely one person suffering the effects of a condition that experts of all backgrounds can't definitively provide a cause or a cure for. That should compel us to humility and empathy for each other. We are all fighting this battle in the dark. Let's walk carefully so we don't knock each other over while we're getting there.

5 FIGHTING THE PAIN

When you face the same or worse levels of pain everyday, it's tempting to stop fighting it. In a society that struggles to face the reality of sustained pain, being a constant reminder of that incurable pain is an awkward position. Communities are great at coming around someone who has just been diagnosed with terminal cancer or someone who's just been through a life-threatening car accident. Meals are provided, and money is donated. People know how to show their compassion for acute conditions. Short-term pain brings out the best in our short-term society.

But what happens when your pain lasts for months or years? How do you cope with pain that makes everyone around you uncomfortable? Sometimes it's just easier to pretend it's not there, because people around you don't want to deal with it. Sometimes it can be tempting to just ignore it or deny it. You might think you can just do what you want and deal with the consequences later, or you might just stop trying to do anything. Why keep trying? Isn't it easier to just accept the limitations the pain has given and stop trying to do things that highlight your newfound weaknesses and pain?

I don't have a "one-size-fits-all" answer. Every situation will call for a potentially different strategy. However, I do feel confident saying this much—pain is something that you must keep fighting. When you decide to give up that fight, you start to lose yourself in the haze of what is going on around you.

A substantial part of that fight consists of owning your pain. In an odd twist, you have to acknowledge and internalize the pain as your own before you can fight it effectively. So what does it mean to own your pain? Should you try to make your pain your new identity? Not exactly. Owning your pain is a feeble attempt at using one word to describe a complicated lifelong process of simultaneously accepting the reality of your pain, while vigorously continuing to fight its control over you on a daily basis. Let's try to break this down a little in a way that's easier to understand.

There are several equally important aspects to owning your pain. The first aspect is accepting the reality of your pain. Trying to live in chronic pain while acting like it doesn't exist will not ultimately solve anything. It will simply accelerate the breakdown of your health and the implosion of your relationships as others try to live with the consequences of your self-destructive choices. In order to effectively own your pain, you must face the reality that it is a part of your life. You didn't want it. You didn't ask for it. You didn't cause it, but it's yours. Now you own it.

At the same time, you must not let the reality of your life of chronic pain stop you from fighting to hold on to the parts of your life that it hasn't stolen. Part of owning your pain is not letting your pain define who you are and what you can do. While you will have to make adjustments in order to function, you will also have to decide where to take a stand.

Once you make that stand, you don't let pain keep you from ever leaving home again or trying something new. For example, you may have to drastically adjust your schedule to manage your limited remaining energy, but that doesn't mean you can never plan to meet up with friends for lunch just because you might be sick that day. You keep making plans, but you make them with the understanding that they may have to change at the last minute.

There are all kinds of limiting decisions that could be passed off as "just being realistic" with the energy you have, but don't let your pain become the ultimate deciding factor. It is simply a part of your decision-making process. It will seem incredibly difficult at first to distinguish between situations where you need to accommodate your pain, and situations where you push through to avoid giving up completely.

I wish I could say that after a while it's easy, but I think it's always going to be a struggle on some level. There will always be some risk when you expend energy. No one who already feels vulnerable likes the thought of risking their paltry amount of energy on something that might not be worth it. But in the long run, the cost of never investing your energy in productive ways is far higher than just making a few unwise decisions in the opposite direction.

To live at all is to accept the fact of risk. Although we may go through phases where we just want to cut off from the world and protect ourselves in a homemade blanket fort, we can't live like that for the rest of our lives. Eventually, we have to come out of our blanket forts and face the decisions of where to spend ourselves.

While it may not ever be easy, it does get somewhat easier when you have plenty of previous experiences to help you make those decisions. You can remember that spending energy on this adventure was worth it for the morale boost, but the physical drain of that task was a total waste. Sadly, you may find that your memory is faulty in detecting these patterns, but having friends and family who can help you keep track of these types of patterns can be an invaluable resource when you are faced with this type of choice.

At some point you can determine what you are willing to spend your energy or "spoons" on, and what isn't worth it *[See "Spoon Theory" at http://www.butyoudontlooksick.com/articles/written-by-christine/the-spoon-theory/]*. The point is not that everyone's lists match up; rather, it is crucial for you to consider your fight against your pain as an individual and strategically choose things that will help you in your fight. Some people will find that holding down a part-time job is a perfect balance to help them keep fighting while accommodating their new limits, but others will have to give up their careers entirely and fill their time with other healthy pursuits. You can't predict what will fill that gap for every person, but everyone will need to fill that activity gap with something.

6 CELEBRATING THE VICTORIES

If you've made it this far, you're probably starting to get a rather dismal view of living with the chronic pain of fibromyalgia. Of course, that's assuming you didn't begin this book already feeling that way about it from your own intimate acquaintance with it. Given the circumstances, it's not hard to see why living with constant, incurable pain could be a miserable existence. It can easily become a very depressing, monotonous cycle of struggle and defeat.

You wind up facing more bad days than good. You see your doctor more often than you see your friends and your pharmacist more than parts of your family. After a while the lifestyle of a chronically ill person can begin to take its toll on even the heartiest person. When this begins to happen, it's vital that you make it a priority to celebrate the victories along the way, even the small ones. Sometimes it might feel silly to celebrate getting out of bed or taking a shower. But in the long run, it can also be therapeutic.

So, what types of victories are we talking about here? Let's discuss some examples. It could be nearly anything; when functioning in normal life is this hard, every moment is a battle at some level. It is within this context that victories show up in the oddest places. You might do a load of laundry in spite of having a bad flare-up. Some days it might be as small and simple as getting out of bed and getting dressed on a day of bad pain.

The size of the victory is not important. What matters is recognizing that even when you are feeling your worst, even when you are struggling to make it through one more day—even then, you are still not failing in every area of your life. When circumstances are tougher than normal, the expectations have to adjust as well. One common reason that many of us within the chronically ill community get so down on ourselves is that we continually push ourselves to our limits. We even push beyond them by comparing our worst flare-up days to healthy days rather than acknowledging the weaknesses and adjusting our expectations to the "new normal." It's true we may not accomplish as much as we would be able to during other weeks, but that doesn't make that accomplishment any less a victory when it's happening.

If we constantly focus on how far we are from being able to do what we once did, or what we think we should be able to do, we are only hurting ourselves. Instead of letting it pull us down into a depressive thought cycle, we could take inventory of our situation and give ourselves some breathing room to allow ourselves room to be hurt, weak, sick, or in pain.

When you realize the obstacles you are facing on a daily basis to simply get out of bed one more time and go on with your life, it helps you to realize that facing a life of chronic pain is a victory all of its own. You don't have to compare your victories to those of people around you. You don't have to measure your life's work against others at work or in your field of expertise or experience. You don't even have to make sure you've achieved your family's expectations for your life. You simply have to live fully with the gifts that God has given you and use them to serve Him to the best of your ability with a grateful heart.

A large part of that process is choosing to focus on the things He has given you the strength to do, the people He keeps in your life, and the roles you are given. You can't afford to let the incredibly hard and painful aspects of your daily existence overshadow the truly beautiful parts.

So it sounds pretty simple and maybe even a bit cliché. Focus on the positive aspects of each day and minimize the negative. Be grateful for what you have instead of comparing it to what others have. Maybe it does sound trite. I can't tell you that it's something I do perfectly or even well on a consistent basis. What I can tell you is that I have found some great strength from celebrating some of the most ridiculously small and insignificant victories. I have had days where I was in tears of joy just because

I'd been able to get dressed and leave our apartment that day after several weeks of hiding from the pain and the rest of the world inside. I've had times where I had to celebrate the fact that I had enough energy to take a shower or go for a walk.

These things may seem small or unimportant, but if you have ever been weak and trapped—unable to process the physical and emotional pain coursing through your body and soul, you will know that these are not small victories. Sometimes they are the very difference between a dark period of depression that drags on for months, and the sun breaking through the clouds with a cool, refreshing breeze.

It's hard to explain unless you've been there, but if you're struggling with the big picture, then I would like you to picture me sitting down across from you. Imagine that I am right there looking you squarely in the eyes, taking your hands, and gently telling you to take it one small, shaky step at a time.

Today, so far, you've chosen life. That gives me hope for you, and that is a victory worth celebrating.

7 INEVITABLE RELAPSE

"If I can just get the right balance of exercise and proper diet..." "If my doctor and I just figure out the right mixture of prescription dosages and rest..." "If, if, if..." There are so many possible ways to pursue your health and wellness when it comes to dealing specifically with fibromyalgia and chronic pain in general.

It's sometimes tempting to believe that if you just get the right combination of whatever you're trying at the moment, you will fix it and never have problems again. Isn't that the fairytale miracle we've all been promised by the commercials and advertising for various forms of treatment regimens? Isn't that what we're secretly promising ourselves as we try one ridiculously restrictive diet after another?

Sadly, the reality is that there is no cure for fibromyalgia and many other chronic conditions that we live with. That means that we are going to have to manage them and deal with them for the rest of our lives. This also means that as restrictive as we get with ourselves and as diligent as we are with following our treatment plans, it is entirely possible and even likely that we will still face temporary setbacks and relapses. In the fibro world we like to call these "flare-ups." These are times when the symptoms of our condition are much worse and more pronounced than they normally would be.

When this happens, it's important to remember that this is not an indication that our treatments have failed or that we have messed up somehow. Even the best treatment plans allow for most patients to still have flare-ups. Perhaps you are one of the few, miraculously fortunate patients who find the perfect combination of medications or therapies and never experience symptoms again. However, for the rest of us who have to deal with flare-ups, it is something that needs to be taken seriously and considered before it happens, so you're ready to deal with it when it comes.nun

Flare-ups can create complications that extend far beyond your original symptoms. Anyone who has made a breakthrough, after suffering through years of trial and error, knows well how devastating that can be emotionally. Enjoying a short respite from pain and fatigue, and falling back into pain after only a few months, is a difficult reality.

You may seem well for several months or even up to a year, or it may only last a few days before you have to deal with the same symptoms again. It can be extremely frustrating and cause you to second guess every health-related decision you've ever made. It can even make it harder to go forward making more decisions, wondering if you're just going to make things worse.

Here's the deal on flare-ups. There really isn't anything that most of us can do to 100% guarantee we will never have another flare-up. It is out of our control. Having said that, there is a pattern among chronically ill people who are starting to get some strength back to push themselves too hard in an attempt to "make up for lost time" by accomplishing a lot while they're feeling well.

Often such overexertion results in a flare-up or a worse than normal flare-up. Then the internal blame game starts. It's natural to feel that you brought the flare-up on yourself from pushing yourself too hard, but ultimately that's not a helpful place to be mentally. Even if there is some truth to the point that you bring some flare-ups on yourself, it does not help you to blame yourself.

Nearly all of us get flare-ups to some degree, and it is a completely normal response to want to work on things while you feel up to it. Sometimes it takes extreme willpower and foresight to stop working before you feel it catching up with you in order to minimize the paralyzing fatigue and pain that will be coming later. Other times, it doesn't matter how early you stop or how careful you are; you will still pay.

We've talked a lot about what you can't do in regard to flare-ups, but what can you do when you're getting a bad flare-up?

There are certain ways to mitigate the effects on your mind, your body, and your emotions so that you are not as beaten down as you might be otherwise.

The next time you feel a flare-up coming on, remember what we've talked about so far. This flare-up is part of your condition. It is something you can handle, and you will. You need to stay calm, keep your head, and avoid blaming yourself for it. Sometimes it's just going to happen.

Another helpful thing to keep in mind when you get your next flare-up is to try to find someone you can discuss it with. Pain is much harder to face alone. Finding a trusted friend or relative who can walk through the rougher, uglier, messier days with you and remind you what your Hope is will be worth its weight in gold. Not every loving person in your life will be a good fit for this role, so it's important to think through this before you're in the middle of a flare-up. Choose your person or people carefully. You won't need very many people, but once you've found them, don't give them up easily.

One possibly obvious suggestion that I will risk making is to treat yourself gently. If you're like most people who spend the majority of their adult lives in pain, you spend a lot of that time feeling frustrated with your limitations and being critical of yourself in order to finish anything.

You are constantly pushing limits to keep up with the rest of society, and sometimes that's what you have to do. But sometimes you need to take it easy when going through a flare-up. There are days when you have to push through, and there are days when you have to lie on the couch and rest. When you have to spend a day on the couch, don't beat yourself up for being weak. Be gentle. You are making a good decision with the resources you have.

One last piece of wisdom that I have learned from my own flare-up experiences the past few years is this. When you are staring your condition in the face and feeling your lowest, remember your ultimate goal. When you're barely able to keep one foot in front of the other and feeling worthless, remember that God does not define your worth by what you can do. Remember why you exist, and thank God for these tangible reminders you can't ignore. Keep your eyes on the prize. This pain won't last forever.

8 LIVING TODAY

I have a bad habit. Well, to be honest, I have many; but the one I'm referring to here is that of dreaming too far ahead. When that happens my feet start to lift off the ground, and I start to lose my grip on the here and now. Sound familiar? This is a part of my personality that I am working on regulating so it doesn't carry me off too much. I have noticed that sometimes it can be a particular liability when it comes to my fibromyalgia. I should be dealing with how the symptoms and side effects are going now. Instead, I am drifting ahead years into the future wondering about my future health and what life will look like down the road as I age with fibromyalgia. I know I am not alone in this fear and obsessing, but I have found that it is not always a helpful place to dwell.

For example, nobody can definitively tell whether someone with fibro will get worse, get better, stay relatively the same, or go back and forth as they get older. It differs with each patient, and that makes things incredibly frustrating at times when trying to look forward. I tend to lean toward the pessimistic side of thinking. I assume that my health will deteriorate as I age, since I can only be pleasantly surprised later on. But when I really stop and think about what I'm doing, it's kind of sad.

I'm 27 right now, and I'm planning the rest of my life around the potential of being very sick and weak physically. This might seem silly to readers joining the conversation from the shores of 50 or 60 who know well the havoc that age can wreak on the human body, but health and disease are topics that are never far away from my mind when planning for the future. My husband and I have been married just slightly over 2 years and we already have felt the need to look into planning out medical power of attorney paperwork. I could argue that it's a good idea for any couple of any age to have such paperwork drawn up to protect their legal interests, but the reality is that it wouldn't even cross my mind if I weren't dealing with this condition. Again, it all comes back to the fibro.

So, what's my point? Am I not supposed to plan ahead? Am I supposed to pretend that I will magically be healed and live a normal life later on? I don't think so. I think planning ahead is important, and I will actually cover that in another chapter. But having said that, I do not think that the present reality should be sacrificed for the sake of what may happen in the future.

The truth is that we have no idea how things are going to go down the road. I may get better, or I might get worse. Either way, we are not there yet. Your condition is much the same if you are dealing with a chronic condition. You can spot trends in different diseases, but ultimately you can't know for sure what your health will be like in the future. I think that is also a gift. Sometimes we are better off not knowing what lies ahead of us.

I am talking about grounding ourselves in what is actually happening. I can't speak for everyone dealing with chronic pain. However, I know from having dealt with it myself for several years nonstop, it can change the way you think about everything. It can make it difficult to live in the present, because you constantly feel threatened and anxious about what may happen in the future.

It's pretty common to find people in this situation who are concerned about losing their jobs due to excessive absences for sick days or feeling too physically drained to even hold down a regular job at all. Even those who are cared for worry about what would happen to them if their families fell on hard times and couldn't provide for them anymore. Mothers and fathers worry about who will provide for their children if their condition prevents them from working or eventually takes them under. It's easy to get caught up in all the things that could go wrong because of this condition and the pain. Just being honest about it—there are lots of things that can go wrong.

I have found that the best way to fight against the overwhelming anxiety and obsession over potential future disasters is to force myself to live in the current reality of today. Yes, I may have long-term goals that may never come true because of my pain and fatigue, but that is not the reality I am living in today. Yes, I may find that my health deteriorates over time, and even coping mechanisms I find helpful now will be unavailable to me down the road. But that is not the situation I am facing right now. Yes, my pain may get much worse and the medications may not be able to handle it sufficiently to allow me to work, but that is not happening today. Yes, I may find that my work-from-home freelancing assignments do not provide enough money and I cannot supplement my husband's income consistently to the degree that I have been, but that is not our current reality.

Our disease can steal a lot from us, but it can steal even more if we allow it to take away our hope. We have to trust that God has just as much power over the future of our condition as He does over the current situation. As hard as it is for those of us who plan and research to obsessive levels (yes, that would include me), sometimes the healthiest option you can choose is to hold your plans with an open hand. You make plans to the best of your ability, and then you leave the results up to God. If He gives the strength and opportunity for this job, or that move, or taking on that project, then I plan to do it. If He lets me get too sick for it, then I'll let it go.

There is so much freedom in holding our relationships, our plans, our hopes, our dreams, and our future with an open hand. The truth is that nobody (not even the healthy people out there) can truly grasp their future plans as a guarantee. You can plan to be healthy and plan to have certain jobs or relationships, but people can be taken away and jobs can be lost. Nothing is guaranteed. We are freed from the constant worry and fear of future loss when we realize this and embrace it, instead of trying to fight for the future we think we deserve.

So if we get all the circumstances we wanted, we will praise God for His mercy over our lives. If we lose everything we held closest and can't even live long enough to see our children grow up, we will still praise Him. We will live in the blessings He's given us today. We will celebrate the victories given to us today, and the future will take care of itself.

9 SHIFTING RELATIONSHIPS

Before I was sick, I had a very narrow view of friendships and relationships. I saw all relationships as something to be entered from a position of strength. I looked for common ground with another person in areas of mutual strength, where we could both look good and benefit each other. It seemed unfathomable that a friendship could include weaknesses.

It was perfectly acceptable to temporarily depend on someone else, but when the time came, you were expected to carry your weight and repay the favor. You could temporarily need help, as long as you were normally self-sufficient. What made my view of this even worse was the fact that I viewed these terms as one-sided. My friends were allowed to need whatever help a normal person might need, but I needed to enter the connection to help, not to constantly need help.

This might sound like an odd arrangement for friendship and when laid out in plain language, it does sound strange and inconsistent. However, this was never presented in such terms; it was just how I viewed things in my head. I suspect I'm not completely alone in these assumptions. When I got sick and could no longer connect on the same levels, I found my views of relationships shifted rather drastically. As I became more active within the online chronic illness community, I have found myself among hundreds of others with the same story.

It seems that many people view friendship as a give-and-take exchange. They are willing to help out their friends on a short-term basis, and they would expect their friends to return the favor within reason. However, when weeks turn into months and the countless bottles of aspirin and heating pads haven't done the trick, patience begins to wear thin. When those friends aren't able to return the normal expectations, some people gradually, politely move on in search of other normal, healthy people.

If you have gone through this transition, you probably already know what I'm talking about. When you begin to slow down because of your condition, your relationships begin to shift—particularly those relationships that depended on you being reliable or consistently available. You might find that people who used to have time for you are no longer available. Friends who used to seem easy to relate to no longer have much in common with you.

Even people who are genuinely caring and compassionate just can't find much to talk about with you anymore, because they don't know how to process the new you. They are the same, but you are a completely new person to them. You are no longer the same person easily defined by work achievements, a busy schedule, a buzzing social life, a hardy family life, or even your talents and life goals. You are now defined, in their eyes at least, by your conditions and limitations. This is sad but too often, still true.

It may take some time to adjust to new perceptions by those around you, but there are also positives to this new stage. In the process of losing old friendships, you may also gain some new ones you never would have had without the pain and fatigue you're facing.

You will probably find that some of your closer friendships are deepened beyond measure as a few people stretch beyond their comfort zone to truly understand what you are going through. They will sit with you in the grieving process of what is gone and start walking with you at a new pace into what is the new reality. The effort made by these precious few will be incomparable, and you will see the beauty and strength of their love and loyalty.

You will also find people that you had no connection with before are now those who understand your pain the best. They can help you navigate the journey ahead because they have been there first. Some of these people may be older and carrying some of the same burdens, but others could be living on the other side of the world—your same age and dealing with the same tough choices you have to make. When each day is an incredible challenge on its own, decisions regarding starting a family or taking a new job become extremely complicated.

It may seem odd to find your friendships turned upside down. You may suddenly realize the people who know you best are those you've only ever met online who share your same condition and symptoms. It will take time for your family to re-learn you, to know how to support you and love you. It will also take time for you to re-learn how to show love and support to your family from your new perspective and situation.

Your pain adds a layer of depth to the fabric of your home, your closest family, and friends. It requires more of everyone, but it also develops strength in you that would not come otherwise. It is hard to explain how being "the sick one" in the group can be a gift. In a way, it prompts you to view people less by how they measure up and makes you more willing to share in their vulnerability.

When my friends who stuck with me through the diagnosis and worst days of unknown symptoms are feeling sick or vulnerable, I can empathize with them. I know they see me as someone well-versed in dealing with pain. When one of my friends is struggling with depression, I can share in their pain and darkness, because I know there are no pretenses to maintain about my own. I am allowed to be close to them in their grief and sorrow, because they know it's safe to take me there.

Relationships like that don't develop by accident, and they don't come out of people showing only their strengths. Relationships like that come from being willing to show your vulnerabilities and trusting that your friends will not judge you for them.

Genuine friendship is a rare gift. Don't begrudge the ones who need to step away when you get sick. Just be so very grateful for the ones who stayed through the worst of it and the new ones who came along to help you keep going.

10 MOVING FORWARD

A lot has been said about chronic illness, both in this book and in others. There is plenty more advice that could be given; if you get online you'll find it in blogs and longer books than this one. There are thousands, perhaps even millions, of people around the world facing fibromyalgia. There are even more within the greater "spoonie" community. If I can take one last chapter to leave you with a parting thought, let it be this one—never stop moving forward. In other words, what happens now? Where do you go from here?

You've been diagnosed. You're trying to get your symptoms under control. You're finding community with others, either through the internet or by the support of people around you. Overall, you seem to be handling the challenges fairly well. So what happens now? You live your life. You make plans, with the understanding that sometimes they will have to be cancelled at the last minute.

You acknowledge that your limits are beyond your control, but sometimes you will push past them. You try to make wise decisions that take your energy and health into account, but you don't beat yourself up if you make the wrong choice. You love everyone else with the love that extends grace instead of expectations. You share your vulnerabilities with those who can appreciate them and build others up in the process.

Having a chronic illness is not the end of your impact on the world. It is merely the entrance to a completely different kind of impact. You will be tempted to think that your weaknesses are liabilities, but they aren't. You may be tempted to see your pain as an obstacle to ministry, but it isn't. And you might wish God had chosen to give your condition to someone else instead, but He didn't. Use the pain God has given you for the one sure purpose you know of—to glorify Him. If that looks like helping others through it, that's great. If it just means trusting Him for the grace to bear it another day, then do it. Grace and peace, my friends.

ABOUT THE AUTHOR

Following a diagnosis of Fibromyalgia in July of 2012, Katie had to make drastic changes to her daily routine. Leaving an enjoyable career as a legal secretary to work from home gave her more flexibility to manage her health, but it wasn't until she started blogging regularly that she began to enjoy sharing her passion for viewing her condition through her faith. This gave birth to the blog, "Walking Through Fog." [www.walkingthroughfog.blogspot.com]

    Since then she has enjoyed sharing pieces of her journey through faith and fatigue with readers as she negotiates her mid-twenties with a life-altering condition. She lives with her husband in a small town in central Indiana where they find love and support from their friends and church family.

Made in the USA
Charleston, SC
02 May 2016